A STROKE
of GRACE

Companion Journal

by

JULIANNE HEAGY

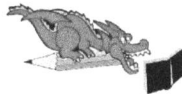

A Wood Dragon Book

A Stroke of Grace - Companion Journal

Cover design: Callum Jagger

Published by:
Wood Dragon Books
Post Office Box 429
Mossbank, Saskatchewan, Canada S0H3G0
www.wooddragonbooks.com

Available in hardcover, paperback, and eBook

978-1-989078-96-9 eBook
978-1-989078-98-3 Hardcover
978-1-989078-99-0 Paperback

Author contact information
Julianne Heagy
Email: AStrokeOfGrace@sasktel.net
Mail: Post Office Box 880, Assiniboia, Saskatchewan, Canada S0H0B0

Facebook: https://www.facebook.com/AStrokeOfGraceByJulianneHeagy
Linktr.ee/AStrokeOfGrace

Dedication

To my husband, Blair, who has been my caregiver, my friend, my confidant, my cheerleader, my rock and the greatest love of my life. Your calm, patience and understanding have made this journey more manageable.

To my dad, Alex Peter, who passed away April 28, 2021. He didn't have the opportunity to see my manuscript turn into a book. I trust he is watching over me and is proud of the work I have done.

To my children, Jared and Justine. Thank you for staying close and for always being loving and supportive—both with this book and life in general. I am so blessed.

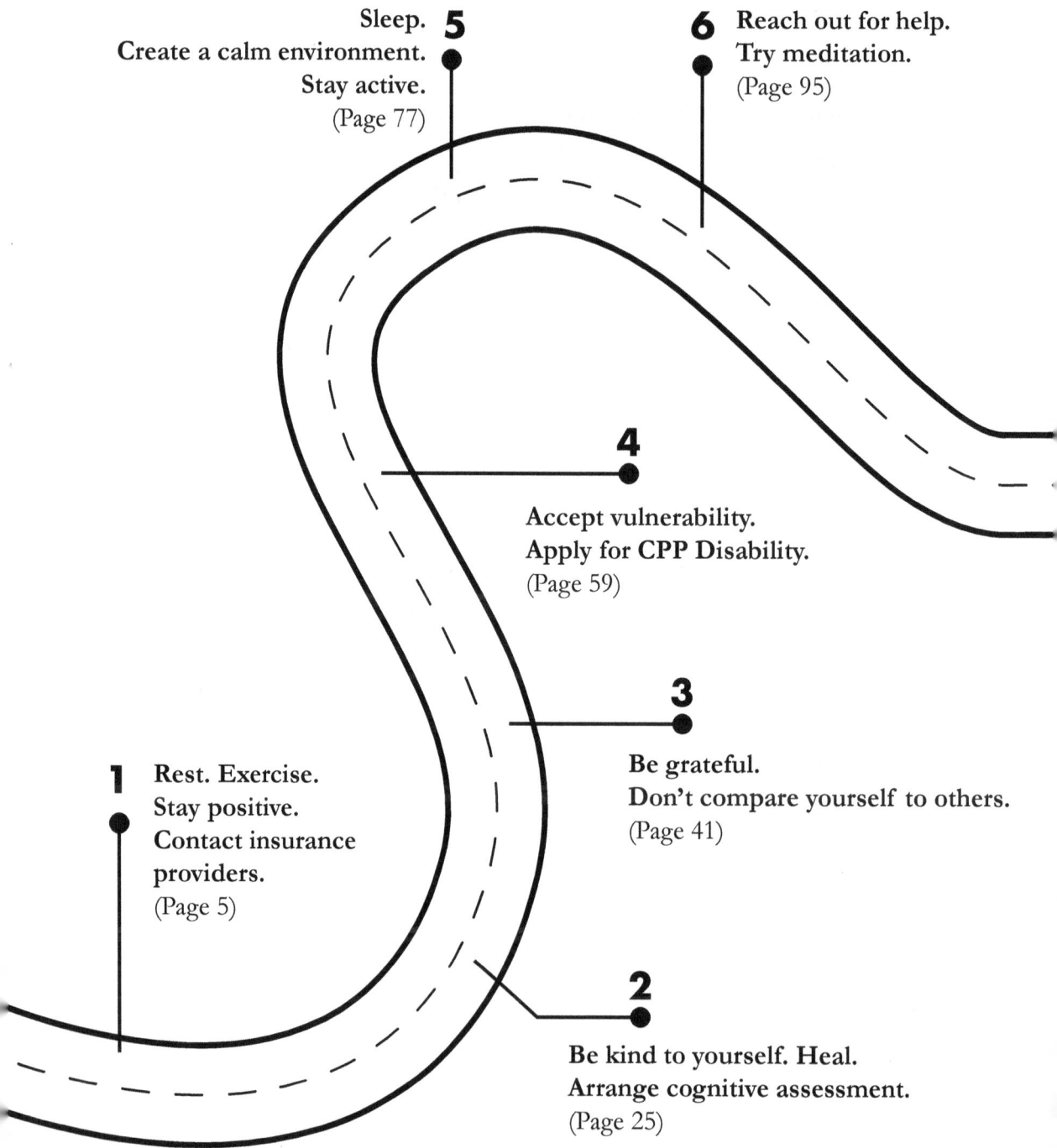

YOUR ROADMAP

5 Sleep.
Create a calm environment.
Stay active.
(Page 77)

6 Reach out for help.
Try meditation.
(Page 95)

4

Accept vulnerability.
Apply for CPP Disability.
(Page 59)

3

Be grateful.
Don't compare yourself to others.
(Page 41)

1 Rest. Exercise.
Stay positive.
Contact insurance
providers.
(Page 5)

2

Be kind to yourself. Heal.
Arrange cognitive assessment.
(Page 25)

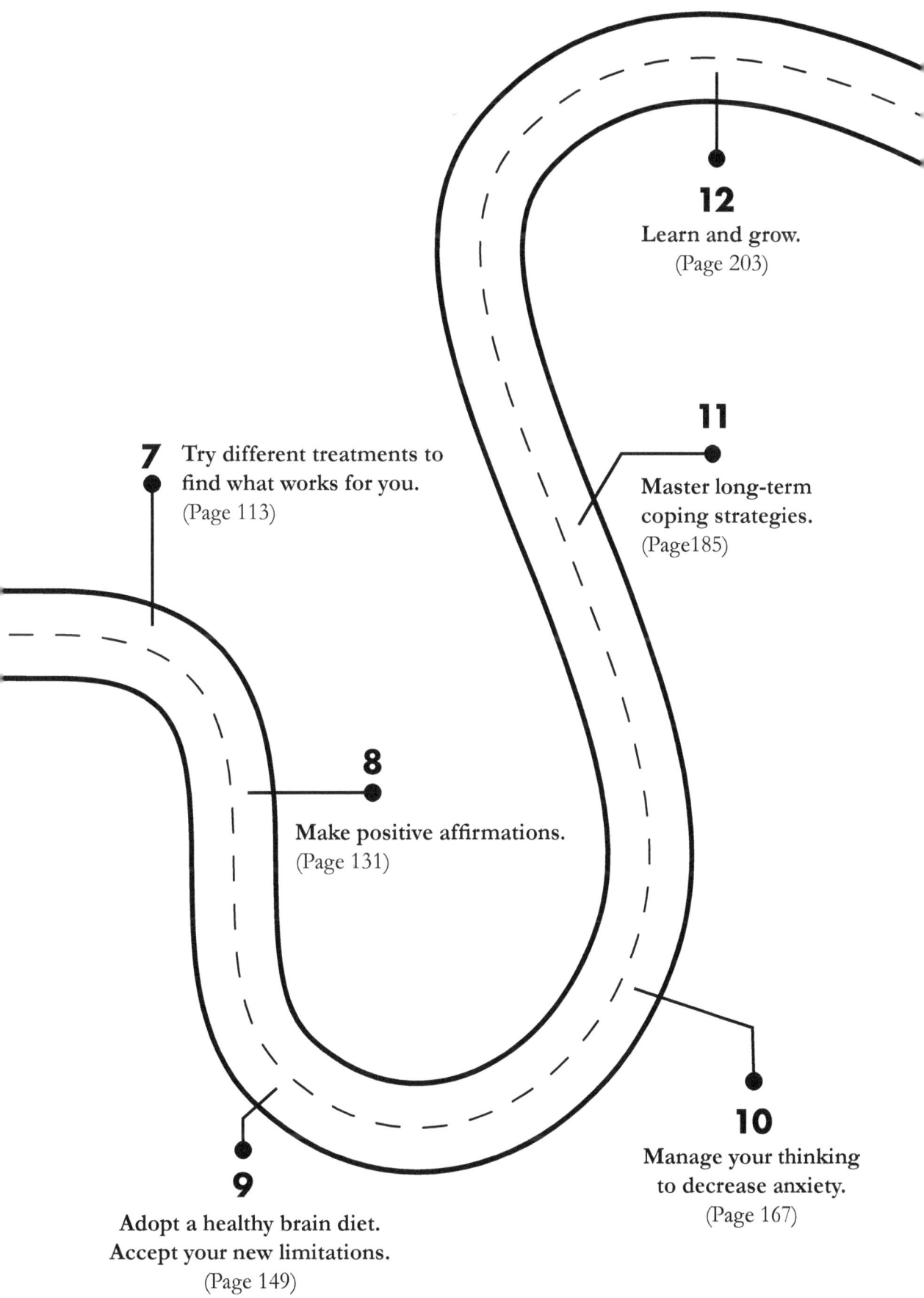

12
Learn and grow.
(Page 203)

11
Master long-term
coping strategies.
(Page185)

7 Try different treatments to
find what works for you.
(Page 113)

8
Make positive affirmations.
(Page 131)

10
Manage your thinking
to decrease anxiety.
(Page 167)

9
Adopt a healthy brain diet.
Accept your new limitations.
(Page 149)

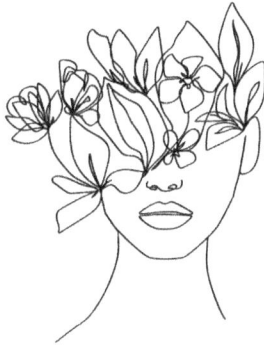

Introduction

During my journey, I discovered that it was easier for me to mentally maneuver if I had all my information in one place; especially when it was time for a medical appointment or to fill out an insurance form. So, I began a journal that documented this vital information, as well as served as a depository for my thoughts and feelings. It had a practical purpose during the year, and at the end of the year, it was a source of affirmation that I had made it! Life had changed forever, but I had made it.

I decided to create this companion journal with a roadmap to help you in your healing journey. It will assist you in keeping track of pertinent medical information and act as a place to reflect on your progress.

This book is arranged in twelve segments, one for each month of the first year after a stroke. Each section begins with "Your Guide and Journey" for that month. Here I share practical tips on maneuvering in your new world, where to find resources, and suggestions on what strategies worked for me to find a place of greater peace and joy within my new limitations.

Following each month's information are pages to document medical appointments. On these pages, there is a section for you to make note of your concerns and questions. This can be used in the days leading up to the appointment. It's not uncommon to leave an appointment and then remember an important concern or question you had hoped to discuss with the practitioner.

Next on the page is space to record appointment dates and times and any other notes such as: *park in the back, bring medication list, do not wear perfume as there is a staff member at the clinic with a perfume allergy.* Also, there is space to record the medical practitioner's contact information. (Insurance providers will ask for this information every time you complete a form, so it is handy to have it all located in one space.)

The "Diagnosis/Advice from Doctor" section is a space to record comments from the doctor/practitioner such as any medication changes or additions, recommended exercises or suggested lifestyle changes.

Following the "Doctor Visit Record" pages, you will find a space to record "Struggles, Successes and Gratitude." This information is especially valuable when you look back and see how far you have come. An example of a "struggle" might be: *headache lasted most of the day, had to stop looking at my computer screen because of visual disturbances, balance seems to be really off this morning.* An example of "success" could be: *slept well, no morning brain fog today, agreed to meet Cathy for coffee and enjoyed a short visit."* (Remember to date your entries.)

Although some days it is hard to find something to be grateful for, it really helps your mental state to dig deep and find something that brings you gratitude. As days pass and you can look back to see an improvement in your "struggles", your gratitude section will have a reason to grow.

The last pages of each segment are pages for journaling. Here you can write down your thoughts and feelings; a private place to express your emotions, ask questions that you hope to find the answers to and/or grow your gratitude practice.

Never in your lifetime will you again experience a year like the year after a stroke. Whether you were the one who survived the stroke or the caregiver, let this book be the roadmap, the information depository, and a safe place for your thoughts.

I wish you well in the year ahead,

Julianne

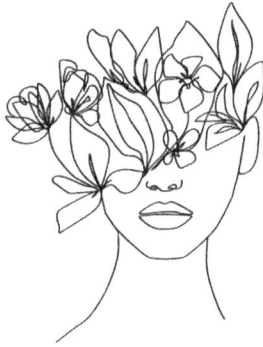

Your Guide and Journey
Month One

Give yourself permission to rest. Your brain has been injured and needs time to heal. Be kind to yourself. The more you push to be on your computer, to read, to push past the fatigue, to carry on with your responsibilities at work, the more you are overstimulating the injured brain. As with any injured body part, there is inflammation. The purpose of inflammation is to tell your body that you're hurt and that you need to rest the injured part to help prevent re-injury.

I know this is hard—especially if you don't have any physical impairment after the stroke. I had a hard time convincing myself I was still "injured"—I couldn't see the damage, nor could friends and family. They assumed I was better because I could walk and talk. I so wanted them to be right.

A stroke is serious business. According to the Journal of Neuroinflammation, *"Stroke is a debilitating disease condition defined as either* *an interruption of blood supply to the brain due to a clot or embolism, or the rupture of a blood vessel in the brain, which then leads to neurological impairments. It remains the 3rd leading cause of death worldwide with nearly 15 million people being affected per year."* [1]

According to the Heart and Stroke Foundation of Canada, *"Stroke is on the rise. Ischemic stroke, caused by a blood clot, occurs in 85% of all stroke patients. A hemorrhagic stroke occurs in the remaining 15% when a blood vessel ruptures, causing bleeding in the brain. A transient ischemic attack (TIA) – sometimes referred to as a mini-stroke – is caused by a small clot that briefly blocks an artery. More than 62,000 strokes occur in Canada each year and that number continues to rise, leaving more than 405,000 people in Canada living with the effect of stroke."* [2]

Being physically able to drive doesn't mean you should. I found out well after the fact that if I had been driving and in a car accident in the first six months following my stroke, I would not have had any insurance coverage. Be sure to check your vehicle insurance for any restrictions you may have.

Reach out to a physiotherapist. Physiotherapists are direct-access practitioners, meaning patients can visit physiotherapists directly (using self-referral) without waiting for a physician referral. [3]

If you haven't already been referred, do yourself a favour and have a physio assessment. You may be unaware of residual weaknesses or imbalances. Now is the time to start your rehabilitation.

When you are approved for physical therapy, don't delay. Retraining the brain and muscles soon after a stroke is very important.

Self-care is vital. Rest, rest, rest. If your anxiety is worse now than it was in the past, it's okay to ask for help and speak with a counsellor.

Learn what works for you; for example, for me, avoiding sugar helps to keep my anxiety down. Know that you have new limitations, as with any injury. Take time to rest and repair.

Avoid self-medicating with drugs and alcohol. Alcohol could interfere with any medicine you take to reduce your risk of having another stroke. In particular, alcohol can be harmful if you are taking blood-thinning medication or if you have had a hemorrhagic stroke. Talk to your doctor about whether it is safe to drink alcohol while taking any medication.

Focus on good nutrition. This is an area you *do* have control over, so help yourself to avoid future strokes. If necessary, search out a nutritionist who can guide you with this. The Heart and Stroke Foundation website is also a great resource.

Exercise within your limits. Falls are a very real risk after a stroke, so walking with a buddy is a great idea.

Stay positive and remain grateful. Some days, you have to "fake it until you make it," especially in these first days. Keep trying to find the things and people you are grateful for. If you have a caregiver, express your awareness of their concern and care. If your caregiver is a family member or friend, remember they are learning about this new life with you.

Find out about Group Long Term Disability. It may be difficult to navigate forms at this point, so find help in obtaining and completing the paperwork necessary to initiate a claim for potential Long Term Disability benefits. In my case, we have a very efficient payroll/benefits administrator at the Co-op office. She explained to me that for the first two weeks after my stroke I would receive sick leave benefits, so my paycheque wouldn't change. Eight days after my stroke, she helped me submit my claim. Our family physician was very quick to complete the Attending Physician's Statement.

On June 26th, I received a letter explaining my benefits would be retroactive back to June 5, and that my income would be 67 percent of my regular monthly salary. It also confirmed that payments would be made by direct deposit and that premiums would be waived for my portion of disability, basic life, and dental insurance through my group policy. It went on to say that my file would be reviewed for rehabilitation opportunities and that regular requests would be made to my doctor for updates on my progress.

It was almost two months after my last paycheque before I received my first, monthly disability payment. This financial strain added to my stress and anxiety.

Use a file folder or some sort of storage container to keep paperwork (such as all your reports, insurance applications, and notes from doctors' appointments) in one place. Don't worry about organizing it right away; hopefully that is a task you'll be able to manage down the road. It's so much easier to fill out the follow-up insurance forms when everything is in one place.

Notes

1   Jayaraj R.L., Azimullah S., Beiram R., Jalal F.Y., Rosenberg G.A. *Neuroinflammation: friend and foe for ischemic stroke. J Neuroinflammation. 2019;16(1):142*

2   *2019 Report on Heart, Stroke and Vascular Impairment.* Heart and Stroke Foundation of Canada. Taken from "(Dis)connected: How unseen links are putting us at risk."

3   According to *physiocanhelp.ca*

DOCTOR VISIT RECORD

Concerns/ Questions

_____

_____

_____

Appointment Details

Date: Time:

Reason for Visit:

_____

Doctor's Details

Name:

Phone:

Address:

Appointment Results

Diagnosis:

_____

Advice from doctor:

_____

Ask your doctor to use this space to note her/his comments regarding this visit:

_____

_____

_____

DOCTOR VISIT RECORD

Concerns/ Questions

_____
_____
_____

Appointment Details

Date: Time:
_____
Reason for Visit:
_____
_____

Doctor's Details

Name:
_____
Phone:
_____
Address:
_____

Appointment Results

Diagnosis:
_____
_____
Advice from doctor:
_____
_____

Ask your doctor to use this space to note her/his comments
regarding this visit:
_____
_____
_____

DOCTOR VISIT RECORD

Concerns/ Questions

Appointment Details

Date: Time:

Reason for Visit:

Doctor's Details

Name:

Phone:

Address:

Appointment Results

Diagnosis:

Advice from doctor:

Ask your doctor to use this space to note her/his comments regarding this visit:

DOCTOR VISIT RECORD

Concerns/ Questions

Appointment Details

Date: Time:

Reason for Visit:

Doctor's Details

Name:

Phone:

Address:

Appointment Results

Diagnosis:

Advice from doctor:

Ask your doctor to use this space to note her/his comments regarding this visit:

DOCTOR VISIT RECORD

Concerns/ Questions

Appointment Details

Date: Time:

Reason for Visit:

Doctor's Details

Name:

Phone:

Address:

Appointment Results

Diagnosis:

Advice from doctor:

Ask your doctor to use this space to note her/his comments regarding this visit:

DOCTOR VISIT RECORD

Concerns/ Questions

Appointment Details

Date: Time:

Reason for Visit:

Doctor's Details

Name:

Phone:

Address:

Appointment Results

Diagnosis:

Advice from doctor:

Ask your doctor to use this space to note her/his comments regarding this visit:

Things I'm grateful for ...

Struggles

Successes

Journal Notes

Journal Notes

Journal Notes

Journal Notes

Journal Notes

Journal Notes

Journal Notes

Journal Notes

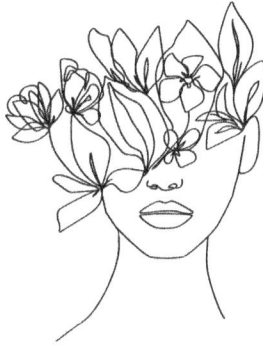

Your Guide and Journey
Month Two

Be kind to yourself and allow yourself time to heal. Take time to rest. Especially for those with cognitive rather than physical impairments, it's hard to not push to get back to "normal." Trust that others who have experienced this have taken a year or more to heal. I know you want to be the exception to that rule. I did.

Limit screen time. At this point in your recovery, you may be bored and want to entertain yourself with video games or checking out your social media. May I suggest a healthier option as suggested to me by the occupational therapist—working on picture puzzles and or handcrafts will not only fill your days, it will keep you from worrying about the future.

Why is it hard on our head to be on a computer screen? According to the Brain Injury Society of Toronto: [1]

- Images that appear on LCD screens are made up of pixels that refresh at a rate of 60 times per second even when the content on the screen is not changing.
- The rapid movement of these pixels means that when we look at screens for too long, we strain our eye muscles.
- For someone who has suffered a brain injury, this strain can be detrimental.
- The backlighting of LCD screens can cause cognitive fatigue, headaches, dizziness, and nausea in brain-injured patients.

Reach out to your local chapter of the Brain Injury Association. In Canada, you can find your closest chapter at: www.braininjurycanada.ca. I often felt that my recovery was my mountain to climb alone. Please know that there is great support through both the provincial chapters and Brain Injury Canada. You'll have an opportunity to meet others with acquired brain injuries and ask questions that make sense to someone else. It is also a great resource for your caregiver to be able to understand what it's like to live with a brain injury.

Find out about your insurance coverage. You've probably already started applying for and maybe even receiving some group benefits through work. I was surprised to find that, because I was over the age of sixty when my stroke occurred, I only had twelve months of long-term disability coverage. Had I been under the age of sixty, my coverage would have been twenty-four months. Insurance coverage varies dramatically with different companies' policies. For example, with my husband's cancer, he has long-term disability benefits until age sixty-five.

At month two, I wasn't able to cognitively work through these policy details, but hopefully your caregiver or someone you trust will be able to help you.

Do you have disability insurance coverage on:

- Your line of credit at the bank?
- Your credit card?
- Your life insurance policies through a waiver of premium rider?

Do you have a critical illness insurance policy? Does it cover stroke?

Canada Pension Plan Disability coverage has a four-month waiting period which we will discuss in "What I have learned …" in chapter four.

Cognitive Assessment. This is an assessment tool completed by occupational therapists, psychiatrists, or neurologists to make a diagnosis and understand a patient's cognitive capabilities. It includes a series of questions and tasks designed to help measure mental functions such as memory, language, and the ability to recognize objects. Some insurance companies require this in order to approve your claim, to determine that you have a cognitive impairment lasting more than thirty days. This is an assessment that should take place in month two of recovery.

Notes

1 Taken in part from the Brain Injury Society of Toronto article: "Reducing screen time post ABI"

DOCTOR VISIT RECORD

Concerns/ Questions

Appointment Details

Date: Time:

Reason for Visit:

Doctor's Details

Name:

Phone:

Address:

Appointment Results

Diagnosis:

Advice from doctor:

Ask your doctor to use this space to note her/his comments regarding this visit:

DOCTOR VISIT RECORD

Concerns/ Questions

Appointment Details

Date: Time:

Reason for Visit:

Doctor's Details

Name:

Phone:

Address:

Appointment Results

Diagnosis:

Advice from doctor:

Ask your doctor to use this space to note her/his comments regarding this visit:

DOCTOR VISIT RECORD

Concerns/Questions

Appointment Details

Date: Time:

Reason for Visit:

Doctor's Details

Name:

Phone:

Address:

Appointment Results

Diagnosis:

Advice from doctor:

Ask your doctor to use this space to note her/his comments regarding this visit:

DOCTOR VISIT RECORD

Concerns/ Questions

Appointment Details

Date: Time:

Reason for Visit:

Doctor's Details

Name:

Phone:

Address:

Appointment Results

Diagnosis:

Advice from doctor:

Ask your doctor to use this space to note her/his comments regarding this visit:

DOCTOR VISIT RECORD

Concerns/ Questions

Appointment Details

Date: Time:

Reason for Visit:

Doctor's Details

Name:

Phone:

Address:

Appointment Results

Diagnosis:

Advice from doctor:

Ask your doctor to use this space to note her/his comments
regarding this visit:

Things I'm grateful for ...

Struggles

Successes

Journal Notes

Journal Notes

Journal Notes

Journal Notes

Journal Notes

Journal Notes

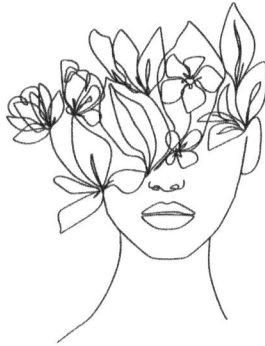

Your Guide and Journey
Month Three

Express and receive gratitude. "When we express gratitude and receive the same, our brain releases dopamine and serotonin, the two crucial neurotransmitters responsible for our emotions, and they make us feel 'good.' They enhance our mood immediately, making us feel happy from the inside." [1]

Remembering to be grateful was a game-changer for me. I didn't make a point of being grateful daily until the end of the first year after my stroke. I wish someone had told me much earlier how very important it is. Expressing gratitude changes your outlook and your perspective.

Consider keeping a daily gratitude journal.

Use resources. If you want to explore the possibility of going back to work, this is a great publication: *Return to Work Following an Acquired Brain Injury. A Self-paced Guidebook and Resources to Help Support You Along* *the Way.* Produced by Brain Injury Canada, it's filled with information such as possible stages of returning to work, reasons for wanting to return to work, establishing a balance, strategies for preparing to leave home (time estimates and planning template), making contact with your employer, pre-return research, workplace policies and employment legislation. There is also a section on learning from others, with personal accounts from people who have gone down this path.

Stop comparing yourself or your situation to others and their situations. In particular, in order to find some peace, I had to stop comparing our financial situation to the circumstances of others. Once I quit thinking about how much we were lacking and started expressing gratitude for what we had, my attitude turned around and I reduced a ton of stress. Albeit, I didn't come across this revelation until almost the end of the first year. I'm hoping that, by sharing this with you now, you won't need to wait that long.

> "Gratitude makes sense of our past, brings peace for today, and creates a vision for tomorrow."
> *Melody Beattie*

> "Gratitude and attitude are not challenges;
> they are choices."
> *Robert Braathe*

Notes

1   The Neuroscience of Gratitude and How It Affects Anxiety & Grief, *PositivePsychology.com,* Jan. 9, 2020

DOCTOR VISIT RECORD

Concerns/ Questions

Appointment Details

Date: Time:

Reason for Visit:

Doctor's Details

Name:

Phone:

Address:

Appointment Results

Diagnosis:

Advice from doctor:

Ask your doctor to use this space to note her/his comments regarding this visit:

DOCTOR VISIT RECORD

Concerns/ Questions

_____

_____

_____

Appointment Details

Date: Time:

Reason for Visit:

_____

Doctor's Details

Name:

Phone:

Address:

Appointment Results

Diagnosis:

_____

Advice from doctor:

_____

Ask your doctor to use this space to note her/his comments regarding this visit:

_____

_____

_____

DOCTOR VISIT RECORD

Concerns/ Questions

Appointment Details

Date: Time:

Reason for Visit:

Doctor's Details

Name:

Phone:

Address:

Appointment Results

Diagnosis:

Advice from doctor:

Ask your doctor to use this space to note her/his comments regarding this visit:

DOCTOR VISIT RECORD

Concerns/Questions

_____
_____
_____
_____

Appointment Details

Date: Time:
_____
Reason for Visit:
_____
_____

Doctor's Details

Name:
_____
Phone:
_____
Address:
_____

Appointment Results

Diagnosis:
_____
_____
Advice from doctor:
_____
_____
Ask your doctor to use this space to note her/his comments
regarding this visit:
_____
_____
_____
_____

DOCTOR VISIT RECORD

Concerns/ Questions

Appointment Details

Date: Time:

Reason for Visit:

Doctor's Details

Name:

Phone:

Address:

Appointment Results

Diagnosis:

Advice from doctor:

Ask your doctor to use this space to note her/his comments regarding this visit:

DOCTOR VISIT RECORD

Concerns/ Questions

Appointment Details

Date: Time:

Reason for Visit:

Doctor's Details

Name:

Phone:

Address:

Appointment Results

Diagnosis:

Advice from doctor:

Ask your doctor to use this space to note her/his comments regarding this visit:

Things I'm grateful for ...

Struggles

_____
_____
_____
_____
_____
_____
_____
_____
_____

Successes

_____
_____
_____
_____
_____
_____
_____
_____
_____
_____
_____

Journal Notes

Journal Notes

Journal Notes

Journal Notes

Journal Notes

Journal Notes

Journal Notes

Journal Notes

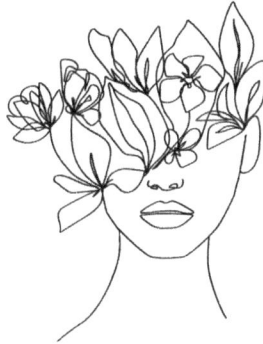

Your Guide and Journey
Month Four

CPP Disability. I include this information about CPP Disability insurance here only because there is usually a four-month waiting period to consider. This is just information to keep in your back pocket until you know it's time to take action. Regardless of what the government website says, pretty much everyone I've spoken with about this has said that from the time they applied to being approved took six to seven months rather than the four-month period suggested on the website. You'll want to keep that in mind if you know that your disability insurance will run out after a year. It's so hard to know at this point if you'll be back to work in six or seven months or if you'll have long-lasting impairments. The link for more information is: https://www.canada.ca/en/services/benefits/publicpensions/cpp/cpp-disability-benefit/apply.html.

The instructions on that website are:

You should apply as soon as you develop a mental or physical condition that:

- prevents you from working regularly at any job
- is long-term and of unknown duration, or is likely to result in death.

Do not delay in sending your completed application form.

Accept vulnerability. I'd explain my fourth month as a period of a little less frustration and maybe a little more vulnerability. I came across this quote from Brené Brown and felt encouraged by it. I hope it encourages you: "Vulnerability is not winning or losing. It's having the courage to show up when you can't control the outcome."

I wish for you the courage it takes to keep showing up. You have what it takes to make your life worth living.

DOCTOR VISIT RECORD

Concerns/ Questions

Appointment Details

Date: Time:

Reason for Visit:

Doctor's Details

Name:

Phone:

Address:

Appointment Results

Diagnosis:

Advice from doctor:

Ask your doctor to use this space to note her/his comments regarding this visit:

DOCTOR VISIT RECORD

Concerns/ Questions

Appointment Details

Date: Time:

Reason for Visit:

Doctor's Details

Name:

Phone:

Address:

Appointment Results

Diagnosis:

Advice from doctor:

Ask your doctor to use this space to note her/his comments regarding this visit:

DOCTOR VISIT RECORD

Concerns/ Questions

Appointment Details

Date: Time:

Reason for Visit:

Doctor's Details

Name:

Phone:

Address:

Appointment Results

Diagnosis:

Advice from doctor:

Ask your doctor to use this space to note her/his comments regarding this visit:

DOCTOR VISIT RECORD

Concerns/ Questions

Appointment Details

Date: Time:

Reason for Visit:

Doctor's Details

Name:

Phone:

Address:

Appointment Results

Diagnosis:

Advice from doctor:

Ask your doctor to use this space to note her/his comments regarding this visit:

DOCTOR VISIT RECORD

Concerns/ Questions

Appointment Details

Date: Time:

Reason for Visit:

Doctor's Details

Name:

Phone:

Address:

Appointment Results

Diagnosis:

Advice from doctor:

Ask your doctor to use this space to note her/his comments regarding this visit:

DOCTOR VISIT RECORD

Concerns/ Questions

_____

_____

_____

Appointment Details

Date: Time:

Reason for Visit:

_____

Doctor's Details

Name:

Phone:

Address:

Appointment Results

Diagnosis:

_____

Advice from doctor:

_____

Ask your doctor to use this space to note her/his comments
regarding this visit:

_____

_____

_____

_____

Things I'm grateful for ...

67

Struggles

Successes

Journal Notes

Journal Notes

Journal Notes

Journal Notes

Journal Notes

Journal Notes

Journal Notes

Journal Notes

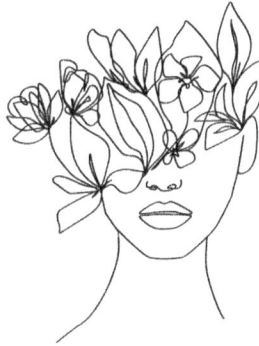

Your Guide and Journey
Month Five

Sleep is vital to your recovery.

According to the neurorehabilitation specialist Henry Hoffman, "Quality sleep has many benefits, especially for stroke survivors. Getting a good night's sleep supports neuroplasticity, the brain's ability to restructure and create new neural connections in healthy parts of the brain, allowing stroke survivors to re-learn movements and functions."

From Hoffman's writings, I learned some tips to improve sleep:

Try to stay consistent in your sleep times – Try to go to bed and wake at the same time each day. A healthy length of sleep is eight hours, so let that be your target.

Avoid daytime naps – I try to avoid naps, but some days it feels like it's not my choice. However, when I don't nap during the day I certainly sleep better at night.

Watch what you eat and drink before bedtime – Avoid overeating before bedtime. In fact, any eating two hours before you go to bed for the night isn't recommended. Caffeine, alcohol, and nicotine are also discouraged late in the day.

Create a calm environment – A room that is cool, quiet, and dark is best. Did you know that research shows that clutter in your space affects anxiety levels, sleep, and the ability to focus? This is a good argument for keeping your bedroom tidy. Video screens really stimulate your brain, so you want to set them aside. If you're not able to read, this would be a good time to listen to an audio book or a sleep meditation until you're ready to sleep.

Address your worries – This might be as simple as having a note pad beside your bed to write down what's on your mind. Once written, set it aside with the intention of dealing with it the next day. I find that deep breathing or any type of meditation is also a good way to settle my mind for the night.

Stay active – Activity is wonderful for encouraging sleep, especially if you can be active outside. (But give yourself a few hours before bedtime as a window to minimize any overly stimulating activities.)

This is a time to draw on our courage and hope. Once we're able to rest, we gain renewed strength and clarity to move on.

> "Perhaps strength doesn't reside in having never been broken but in the courage required to grow strong in the broken places."
> – *Necole Stephens*

DOCTOR VISIT RECORD

Concerns/ Questions

Appointment Details

Date: Time:

Reason for Visit:

Doctor's Details

Name:

Phone:

Address:

Appointment Results

Diagnosis:

Advice from doctor:

Ask your doctor to use this space to note her/his comments regarding this visit:

DOCTOR VISIT RECORD

Concerns/ Questions

Appointment Details

Date: Time:

Reason for Visit:

Doctor's Details

Name:

Phone:

Address:

Appointment Results

Diagnosis:

Advice from doctor:

Ask your doctor to use this space to note her/his comments regarding this visit:

DOCTOR VISIT RECORD

Concerns/Questions

Appointment Details

Date: Time:

Reason for Visit:

Doctor's Details

Name:

Phone:

Address:

Appointment Results

Diagnosis:

Advice from doctor:

Ask your doctor to use this space to note her/his comments regarding this visit:

DOCTOR VISIT RECORD

Concerns/ Questions

Appointment Details

Date: Time:

Reason for Visit:

Doctor's Details

Name:

Phone:

Address:

Appointment Results

Diagnosis:

Advice from doctor:

Ask your doctor to use this space to note her/his comments regarding this visit:

DOCTOR VISIT RECORD

Concerns/ Questions

Appointment Details

Date: Time:

Reason for Visit:

Doctor's Details

Name:

Phone:

Address:

Appointment Results

Diagnosis:

Advice from doctor:

Ask your doctor to use this space to note her/his comments regarding this visit:

DOCTOR VISIT RECORD

Concerns/ Questions

Appointment Details

Date: Time:

Reason for Visit:

Doctor's Details

Name:

Phone:

Address:

Appointment Results

Diagnosis:

Advice from doctor:

Ask your doctor to use this space to note her/his comments regarding this visit:

Things I'm grateful for ...

Struggles

Successes

Journal Notes

Journal Notes

Journal Notes

Journal Notes

Journal Notes

Journal Notes

Journal Notes

Journal Notes

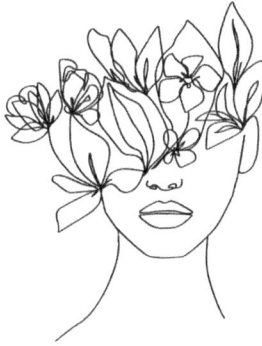

Your Guide and Journey
Month Six

Reach out for help. This was a hard lesson to learn. I've always been a take-charge kinda gal, so reaching out doesn't come easy for me. I'm so relieved for the help when I do finally reach out. I was so grateful for the Acquired Brain Injury support group, and the physiotherapists who provided such helpful information. Although we can easily get caught up in our own world of recovery, it's important to not get so focused on our own suffering and worry that we are unable to see there are times we need to ask for help.

I feel like reaching out is a sign of weakness, but I have learned that it truly is an act of courage and strength. Be open to blessing those around you with the opportunity to make your life a little easier.

Consider sleep meditation. There is a lot of science behind how meditation can help lay down new brain pathways. In an audio book I found helpful, *Meditations to Change Your Brain*, Rick Hanson, PhD, and Richard Mendius, MD report how meditation can help reduce cortisol, the hormone associated with stress. In the studies, meditation increased the natural melatonin levels to help with more restful sleep. It can also encourage greater focus, emotional control, and thoughtful decision making.

The sleep meditations I listened to are Dauchsy Sleep Meditations. I have to say I was a little distrusting at first; I was naively afraid that maybe someone talking to me in my sleep could put the suggestion in my head that robbing a bank was okay, or something similarly bizarre. What I found, after listening, was that I had markedly increased quality and quantity of sleep. The topics are varied in the Dauchsy series; for example, they cover gratitude, healing, creativity, love attraction, and prosperity. (I definitely feel that I have greater peace of mind and feel more optimistic during the day after having listened to a sleep meditation. I find that the sleep meditations lasting no longer than two hours are the best for me, for some reason. Longer ones seem to always wake me at some point, and then I have a hard time getting back to sleep. I continue to listen to sleep meditations three to four nights a week).

"Be strong enough to stand alone, smart enough to know when you need help, and brave enough to ask for it."
Author unknown

"Don't be shy about asking for help. It doesn't mean you're weak, it only means you're wise."
Author unknown

DOCTOR VISIT RECORD

Concerns/ Questions

Appointment Details

Date: Time:

Reason for Visit:

Doctor's Details

Name:

Phone:

Address:

Appointment Results

Diagnosis:

Advice from doctor:

Ask your doctor to use this space to note her/his comments regarding this visit:

DOCTOR VISIT RECORD

Concerns/ Questions

Appointment Details

Date: Time:

Reason for Visit:

Doctor's Details

Name:

Phone:

Address:

Appointment Results

Diagnosis:

Advice from doctor:

Ask your doctor to use this space to note her/his comments regarding this visit:

DOCTOR VISIT RECORD

Concerns/ Questions

Appointment Details

Date: Time:

Reason for Visit:

Doctor's Details

Name:

Phone:

Address:

Appointment Results

Diagnosis:

Advice from doctor:

Ask your doctor to use this space to note her/his comments regarding this visit:

DOCTOR VISIT RECORD

Concerns/ Questions

Appointment Details

Date: Time:

Reason for Visit:

Doctor's Details

Name:

Phone:

Address:

Appointment Results

Diagnosis:

Advice from doctor:

Ask your doctor to use this space to note her/his comments regarding this visit:

DOCTOR VISIT RECORD

Concerns/ Questions

Appointment Details

Date: Time:

Reason for Visit:

Doctor's Details

Name:

Phone:

Address:

Appointment Results

Diagnosis:

Advice from doctor:

Ask your doctor to use this space to note her/his comments regarding this visit:

DOCTOR VISIT RECORD

Concerns/ Questions

Appointment Details

Date: Time:

Reason for Visit:

Doctor's Details

Name:

Phone:

Address:

Appointment Results

Diagnosis:

Advice from doctor:

Ask your doctor to use this space to note her/his comments regarding this visit:

Things I'm grateful for ...

Struggles

Successes

Journal Notes

Journal Notes

Journal Notes

Journal Notes

Journal Notes

Journal Notes

Journal Notes

Journal Notes

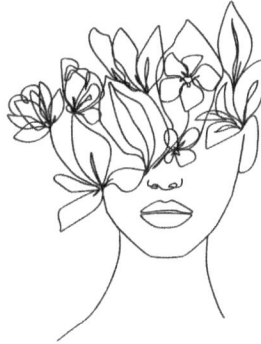

Your Guide and Journey
Month Seven

Are you missing reading? Audiobooks and podcasts are a wonderful way to "scratch that itch." There are lots of free apps to help you. I use the "Libby" app, which is tied to our local library. There are still so many questions I have about my brain's ability to heal. I've listened to Dr. Daniel Amen speak in a few podcasts and have found him to be both encouraging and informative. In his research, he has connected mental health issues to brain injuries. In podcasts, he discusses how researchers are finding new ways to heal the brain and resolve countless numbers of symptoms.

Be aware that you may be required to have cognitive assessments for insurance or other reasons. The testing I had to do is not a usual requirement for all claimants. However, it is important to be aware that further testing may be required to approve your claim.

Try different treatments to find what works for you. My research found the following benefits of Indian Head Massage:

- Helps prevent migraines, headaches, and back pain
- Relieves sleeplessness, restlessness, and insomnia (I can confirm that this treatment helped my sleep the afternoon, night, and for four or five days following the treatment.)
- Relieves symptoms of anxiety and depression (It definitely had a calming effect on me.)
- Renews energy levels
- Boosts memory capabilities (This was not noticeable for me but may increase with regular treatments.)

Create the highest, grandest vision possible for your life, because you become what you believe.
Oprah Winfrey

DOCTOR VISIT RECORD

Concerns/ Questions

Appointment Details

Date: Time:

Reason for Visit:

Doctor's Details

Name:

Phone:

Address:

Appointment Results

Diagnosis:

Advice from doctor:

Ask your doctor to use this space to note her/his comments regarding this visit:

DOCTOR VISIT RECORD

Concerns/ Questions

Appointment Details

Date: Time:

Reason for Visit:

Doctor's Details

Name:

Phone:

Address:

Appointment Results

Diagnosis:

Advice from doctor:

Ask your doctor to use this space to note her/his comments regarding this visit:

DOCTOR VISIT RECORD

Concerns/ Questions

Appointment Details

Date: Time:

Reason for Visit:

Doctor's Details

Name:

Phone:

Address:

Appointment Results

Diagnosis:

Advice from doctor:

Ask your doctor to use this space to note her/his comments regarding this visit:

DOCTOR VISIT RECORD

Concerns/ Questions

_____
_____
_____

Appointment Details

Date: Time:
_____

Reason for Visit:
_____
_____

Doctor's Details

Name:
_____

Phone:
_____

Address:
_____

Appointment Results

Diagnosis:
_____
_____

Advice from doctor:
_____
_____

Ask your doctor to use this space to note her/his comments regarding this visit:
_____
_____
_____

DOCTOR VISIT RECORD

Concerns/ Questions

Appointment Details

Date: Time:

Reason for Visit:

Doctor's Details

Name:

Phone:

Address:

Appointment Results

Diagnosis:

Advice from doctor:

Ask your doctor to use this space to note her/his comments regarding this visit:

DOCTOR VISIT RECORD

Concerns/ Questions

Appointment Details

Date: Time:

Reason for Visit:

Doctor's Details

Name:

Phone:

Address:

Appointment Results

Diagnosis:

Advice from doctor:

Ask your doctor to use this space to note her/his comments regarding this visit:

Things I'm grateful for ...

Struggles

Successes

Journal Notes

Journal Notes

Journal Notes

Journal Notes

Journal Notes

Journal Notes

Journal Notes

Journal Notes

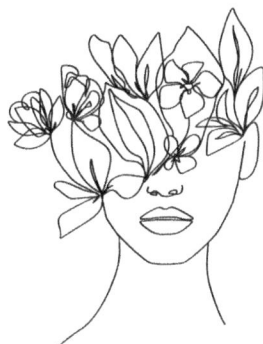

Your Guide and Journey
Month Eight

What you focus on grows. I am understanding that idea more and more. It's as easy, and as hard, as changing your attitude about how you perceive what's going on in your life. For me, I had to consciously quit thinking that we lacked finances. Instead, when those thoughts crept in, I would make a point of being grateful for our safe, comfortable home or the food in our fridge and freezer, or the warmth of our bed. The less time I spent stewing about our financial shortfalls, the more it seemed that money came our way and stayed with us longer.

I also kept hearing myself tell people what I couldn't do. I made a conscious effort to change that conversation to celebrating what I could do. I can listen to audio books and podcasts to scratch that itch I have to learn and enjoy a good story being told. I reveled in telling about the wonderful meals we'd been cooking at home. After all, with my side business of selling cookware, I had a wonderfully stocked kitchen of great cooking tools and really enjoyed spending time creating new dishes. I even began talking about writing a book, trusting that what I focused on would grow.

Make positive affirmations. They help to keep you in a clear, constructive frame of mind. We all have negative beliefs about ourselves. Making positive affirmations is a great way to change that programming in our thoughts to help us feel better about ourselves and where we are in life. Some days I need to tell myself that I'm okay and that I'm not broken. I allow myself to think, *What if I wasn't broken? What could I do? What can I do? What can I be?* I believe that all things happen for good even if that means going through a hard space to find out what that is. Some days I have to dig deep past the frustration and fear and give myself permission to be happily retired and to be grateful for the days I get to spend hanging out with Blair.

Take a moment to think about what you are currently believing about yourself. Awareness is the first step. The trick is to say these positive affirmations consistently, even if you don't believe them at first. The subconscious mind is powerful. We just need to feed it the right information—the right beliefs for our lives.

Write your affirmations in the positive, using "I am" statements. State your declaration in the present tense and include emotion words such as *enjoy, grateful for, excited about, enthusiastic about,* and *focused on.*

Here are a few of mine:

I am strong enough.
I am grateful to be able to write and share my story to help others. I give myself permission to be a successful, inspired writer/author/speaker.
I am able to encourage, empower, and educate stroke survivors and their caregivers.
I am obediently following God's path and purpose for me.

I am compassionate.

I am financially abundant. Money flows to me easily, freely, and abundantly.

I am filled with God's love and joy to overflowing.

I am worthy.

I love and forgive myself.

DOCTOR VISIT RECORD

Concerns/ Questions

Appointment Details

Date: Time:

Reason for Visit:

Doctor's Details

Name:

Phone:

Address:

Appointment Results

Diagnosis:

Advice from doctor:

Ask your doctor to use this space to note her/his comments regarding this visit:

DOCTOR VISIT RECORD

Concerns/ Questions

Appointment Details

Date: Time:

Reason for Visit:

Doctor's Details

Name:

Phone:

Address:

Appointment Results

Diagnosis:

Advice from doctor:

Ask your doctor to use this space to note her/his comments regarding this visit:

DOCTOR VISIT RECORD

Concerns/ Questions

Appointment Details

Date: Time:

Reason for Visit:

Doctor's Details

Name:

Phone:

Address:

Appointment Results

Diagnosis:

Advice from doctor:

Ask your doctor to use this space to note her/his comments regarding this visit:

DOCTOR VISIT RECORD

Concerns/ Questions

Appointment Details

Date: Time:

Reason for Visit:

Doctor's Details

Name:

Phone:

Address:

Appointment Results

Diagnosis:

Advice from doctor:

Ask your doctor to use this space to note her/his comments regarding this visit:

DOCTOR VISIT RECORD

Concerns/ Questions

Appointment Details

Date: Time:

Reason for Visit:

Doctor's Details

Name:

Phone:

Address:

Appointment Results

Diagnosis:

Advice from doctor:

Ask your doctor to use this space to note her/his comments regarding this visit:

Things I'm grateful for ...

Struggles

Successes

Journal Notes

Journal Notes

Journal Notes

Journal Notes

Journal Notes

Journal Notes

Journal Notes

Journal Notes

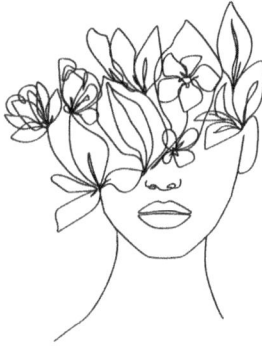

Your Guide and Journey
Month Nine

Learn about the role of diet in your brain health. There is so much we can do to help our brain just by paying attention to the food we eat. The brain uses about 20 to 30 percent of our energy intake. Eating a diet that contains brain-healthy nutrients is essential for good brain health.

The following are some brain-healthy foods you can add to your diet. Or take a moment now and celebrate the good you're already doing!

- Fatty fish (tuna, herring, sardines) are a high source of omega-3 fatty acids, a building block for the brain. Omega-3 helps sharpen memory and improve mood. It may also protect your brain against cognitive decline.
- Blueberries are rich in antioxidants and also have an anti-inflammatory property. They may delay brain aging and improve memory.

- Turmeric has curcumin as its active ingredient. Curcumin has been shown to cross the blood-brain barrier to benefit the brain cells with improved memory, ease of depression and new brain cell growth. You can buy curcumin as a supplement, as the percentage available in turmeric is quite low.
- Broccoli also has antioxidants which may help protect the brain against damage. Broccoli is also very high in Vitamin K. Some studies link Vitamin K to better memory and cognitive status.
- Dark chocolate is packed with brain-boosting compounds such as flavonoids (antioxidant, anti-inflammatory, and immune-boosting), caffeine, and antioxidants (Halleluia!). According to research, chocolate is also a mood booster.
- Some studies show that sage enhances memory.

Listen to your thoughts about other people. If they are negative thoughts, stop them and replace them with thoughts of what you appreciate about that person. I find this particularly helpful as our family relationships are changing. If my filters are less effective at keeping my thoughts to myself, I want to be sharing positive thoughts. This all takes practice, but is worth the effort.

DOCTOR VISIT RECORD

Concerns/ Questions

_____

_____

_____

Appointment Details

Date: Time:

Reason for Visit:

_____

Doctor's Details

Name:

Phone:

Address:

Appointment Results

Diagnosis:

_____

Advice from doctor:

_____

Ask your doctor to use this space to note her/his comments
regarding this visit:

_____

_____

DOCTOR VISIT RECORD

Concerns/ Questions

Appointment Details

Date: Time:

Reason for Visit:

Doctor's Details

Name:

Phone:

Address:

Appointment Results

Diagnosis:

Advice from doctor:

Ask your doctor to use this space to note her/his comments regarding this visit:

DOCTOR VISIT RECORD

Concerns/Questions

Appointment Details

Date: Time:

Reason for Visit:

Doctor's Details

Name:

Phone:

Address:

Appointment Results

Diagnosis:

Advice from doctor:

Ask your doctor to use this space to note her/his comments regarding this visit:

DOCTOR VISIT RECORD

Concerns/ Questions

Appointment Details

Date: Time:

Reason for Visit:

Doctor's Details

Name:

Phone:

Address:

Appointment Results

Diagnosis:

Advice from doctor:

Ask your doctor to use this space to note her/his comments regarding this visit:

DOCTOR VISIT RECORD

Concerns/ Questions

Appointment Details

Date: Time:

Reason for Visit:

Doctor's Details

Name:

Phone:

Address:

Appointment Results

Diagnosis:

Advice from doctor:

Ask your doctor to use this space to note her/his comments regarding this visit:

DOCTOR VISIT RECORD

Concerns/ Questions

Appointment Details

Date: Time:

Reason for Visit:

Doctor's Details

Name:

Phone:

Address:

Appointment Results

Diagnosis:

Advice from doctor:

Ask your doctor to use this space to note her/his comments regarding this visit:

Things I'm grateful for ...

Struggles

Successes

Journal Notes

Journal Notes

Journal Notes

Journal Notes

Journal Notes

Journal Notes

Journal Notes

Journal Notes

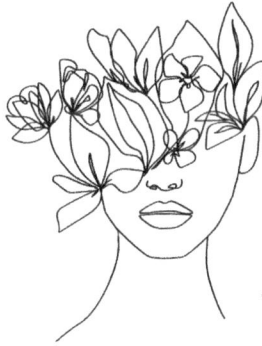

Your Guide and Journey
Month Ten

Try this exercise to decrease anxiety. Whether it's a pandemic or any other life event that is causing anxiety, here is an exercise that will keep everything in perspective. When anxious thoughts are running through your mind, write them down. It might look like this:

- "I'm going to die. My kids are going to die!"
- "I can't work. I have no income! I'm going to be bankrupt!"
- "I'm so scared. Is this literally going to be the end of the world?"

Now, are these thoughts/statements *true*? Do a little research; it'll make you feel better.

- Why are you worrying about death right now? What are some statistics about death? Is the death rate low in your area? Check the rates for the age groups that apply to you or your family.

- Are there other work options that will make you feel safer? Working from home? Different job? When you feel that you're in a financial crisis, it's a good time to look at your spending habits. Living through a pandemic makes you realize that you *can* live without movies, pub nights with friends, vacations to faraway destinations. If you can cut back enough to reduce your stress, even for a short time or even a year or two, you will find your financial footing again. Don't hesitate to reach out for help from financial advisors. They are wonderful at helping you see the truth of your situation rather than live in fear.
- No matter the gravity of the situation, like the pandemic, really think about it. Is it the end of the world? Who knows? If it were, is there anything you can do to change it? Instead of spending your days in fear, open your heart and eyes to the blessings in your life. You have so much to be grateful for. This is a great time to hold firm to your faith, your higher power, your love for one another.

DOCTOR VISIT RECORD

Concerns/ Questions

Appointment Details

Date: Time:

Reason for Visit:

Doctor's Details

Name:

Phone:

Address:

Appointment Results

Diagnosis:

Advice from doctor:

Ask your doctor to use this space to note her/his comments regarding this visit:

DOCTOR VISIT RECORD

Concerns/ Questions

Appointment Details

Date: Time:

Reason for Visit:

Doctor's Details

Name:

Phone:

Address:

Appointment Results

Diagnosis:

Advice from doctor:

Ask your doctor to use this space to note her/his comments regarding this visit:

DOCTOR VISIT RECORD

Concerns/ Questions

Appointment Details

Date: Time:

Reason for Visit:

Doctor's Details

Name:

Phone:

Address:

Appointment Results

Diagnosis:

Advice from doctor:

Ask your doctor to use this space to note her/his comments regarding this visit:

DOCTOR VISIT RECORD

Concerns/ Questions

Appointment Details

Date: Time:

Reason for Visit:

Doctor's Details

Name:

Phone:

Address:

Appointment Results

Diagnosis:

Advice from doctor:

Ask your doctor to use this space to note her/his comments regarding this visit:

DOCTOR VISIT RECORD

Concerns/ Questions

Appointment Details

Date: Time:

Reason for Visit:

Doctor's Details

Name:

Phone:

Address:

Appointment Results

Diagnosis:

Advice from doctor:

Ask your doctor to use this space to note her/his comments regarding this visit:

DOCTOR VISIT RECORD

Concerns/ Questions

_____

_____

_____

Appointment Details

Date: Time:

Reason for Visit:

Doctor's Details

Name:

Phone:

Address:

Appointment Results

Diagnosis:

Advice from doctor:

Ask your doctor to use this space to note her/his comments regarding this visit:

_____

_____

_____

Things I'm grateful for ...

Struggles

Successes

Journal Notes

Journal Notes

Journal Notes

Journal Notes

Journal Notes

Journal Notes

Journal Notes

Journal Notes

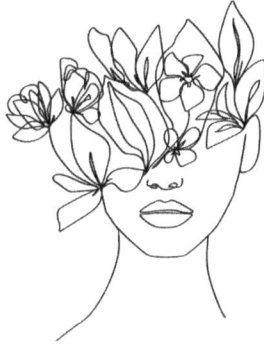

Your Guide and Journey
Month Eleven

Learn about CPP Disability Benefits. It's hard to know when to apply for CPP Disability. You want to believe that tasks will get easier, that you won't always feels so limited, that you'll get back to the old you and the old job, but, in reality, you need to consider your financial future.

Prepare to give the process lots of time. In the end, my application took seven months to approve. This could be because Covid affected so many jobs, including people transitioning to working from home, or delays in mail delivery and processing paperwork.

I found that once my application was approved, I was encouraged to take training if I felt I could work in another career. There is a set gross income you are allowed to earn without affecting your benefits. For the year I was first approved, it was $5,900 per year. I was encouraged by this. I feel that, after Covid, I might want to find some part-time work or maybe even try to work my home business again. Unlike the insurance coverage on our line of credit, which threatens to terminate coverage if I have any income at all, CPP encourages some back-to-work efforts.

One CPP rep told me that if I want to try to go back to work, but then find that I'm unable to do so, that my coverage will be reinstated without the long application process that I started with.

If you have access to a financial advisor, this would be a great time to have a discussion and receive some guidance.

Find coping strategies for anxiety. My anxiety was worse after my stroke. Add a pandemic to the normal stressors of life and we can all use some coping strategies for our anxiety. Here are a few I found helpful.

- Watch a funny video—laughter really is the best medicine.
- Eat well-balanced meals and avoid sugar.
- Limit alcohol and caffeine, which can aggravate anxiety and trigger panic attacks.
- Get enough sleep (see tips on how to get a good night's sleep in Chapter 5).
- Exercise daily to help you feel good and maintain your health—remember that any activity that increases your heart rate and requires you to breathe more often will bring extra oxygen to your brain, and that's a good thing!
- Take deep breaths—inhale slowly and deeply through your nose. Keep your shoulders relaxed. Exhale slowly through your mouth with lips pursed and jaw relaxed. Repeat until you feel more relaxed. Deep breathing counteracts the fight or flight stress reaction.

- Count to 10 slowly. Mostly, this will help bring your attention to the present moment.
- Practice the 5-4-3-2-1 Grounding Technique—This will help manage your anxiety by anchoring yourself in the present. Start by looking for 5 things you can see; become aware of 4 things you can touch; acknowledge 3 things you can hear; notice 2 things you can smell; then, become aware of 1 thing you can taste.
- Use meditation, especially sleep meditation. Not only does it improve sleep, you may experience the following outcomes: waking rested and calm, fewer headaches, lower blood pressure, reduced memory loss, and relief from depression and anxiety.
- Turn to prayer. Remember where your strength lies.

DOCTOR VISIT RECORD

Concerns/ Questions

_____

_____

_____

Appointment Details

Date: Time:

Reason for Visit:

_____

Doctor's Details

Name:

Phone:

Address:

Appointment Results

Diagnosis:

_____

Advice from doctor:

_____

Ask your doctor to use this space to note her/his comments regarding this visit:

_____

_____

_____

DOCTOR VISIT RECORD

Concerns/ Questions

Appointment Details

Date: Time:

Reason for Visit:

Doctor's Details

Name:

Phone:

Address:

Appointment Results

Diagnosis:

Advice from doctor:

Ask your doctor to use this space to note her/his comments regarding this visit:

DOCTOR VISIT RECORD

Concerns/Questions

Appointment Details

Date: Time:

Reason for Visit:

Doctor's Details

Name:

Phone:

Address:

Appointment Results

Diagnosis:

Advice from doctor:

Ask your doctor to use this space to note her/his comments regarding this visit:

DOCTOR VISIT RECORD

Concerns/ Questions

Appointment Details

Date: Time:

Reason for Visit:

Doctor's Details

Name:

Phone:

Address:

Appointment Results

Diagnosis:

Advice from doctor:

Ask your doctor to use this space to note her/his comments regarding this visit:

DOCTOR VISIT RECORD

Concerns/ Questions

Appointment Details

Date: Time:

Reason for Visit:

Doctor's Details

Name:

Phone:

Address:

Appointment Results

Diagnosis:

Advice from doctor:

Ask your doctor to use this space to note her/his comments regarding this visit:

Things I'm grateful for ...

Struggles

Successes

Journal Notes

Journal Notes

Journal Notes

Journal Notes

Journal Notes

Journal Notes

Journal Notes

Journal Notes

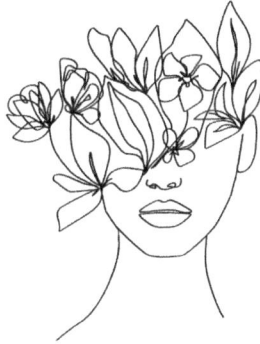

Your Guide and Journey
Month Twelve

Do all you can to continue to learn and grow. If you're unable to read, tune into motivational and/or educational webinars. If looking at monitors bothers your head, tune into podcasts and audio books. There is so much wisdom out there that can guide us to living the best life we can, brain injury or not, regardless of our circumstances.

Acceptance of your post-brain injury abilities will help to protect your quality of life. Dwelling, in a negative way, on limitations you now experience can become overwhelming. Push yourself to focus on what you *can* do and grow from there.

DOCTOR VISIT RECORD

Concerns/ Questions

_____

_____

_____

Appointment Details

Date: Time:

Reason for Visit:

Doctor's Details

Name:

Phone:

Address:

Appointment Results

Diagnosis:

_____

Advice from doctor:

_____

Ask your doctor to use this space to note her/his comments regarding this visit:

_____

_____

_____

DOCTOR VISIT RECORD

Concerns/ Questions

Appointment Details

Date: Time:

Reason for Visit:

Doctor's Details

Name:

Phone:

Address:

Appointment Results

Diagnosis:

Advice from doctor:

Ask your doctor to use this space to note her/his comments regarding this visit:

DOCTOR VISIT RECORD

Concerns/Questions

Appointment Details

Date: Time:

Reason for Visit:

Doctor's Details

Name:

Phone:

Address:

Appointment Results

Diagnosis:

Advice from doctor:

Ask your doctor to use this space to note her/his comments regarding this visit:

DOCTOR VISIT RECORD

Concerns/ Questions

Appointment Details

Date: Time:

Reason for Visit:

Doctor's Details

Name:

Phone:

Address:

Appointment Results

Diagnosis:

Advice from doctor:

Ask your doctor to use this space to note her/his comments regarding this visit:

DOCTOR VISIT RECORD

Concerns/ Questions

Appointment Details

Date: Time:

Reason for Visit:

Doctor's Details

Name:

Phone:

Address:

Appointment Results

Diagnosis:

Advice from doctor:

Ask your doctor to use this space to note her/his comments regarding this visit:

Things I'm grateful for ...

Struggles

Successes

Journal Notes

Journal Notes

Journal Notes

Journal Notes

Journal Notes

Journal Notes

Journal Notes

Journal Notes

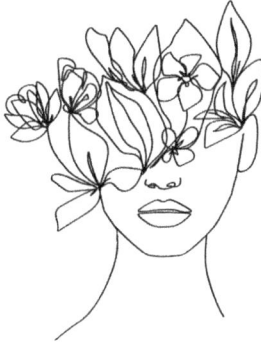

Final Thoughts

As I complete the writing of this book, I'm happy to write that I'm in a space of greater joy and peace.

What have I learned through this experience that I really want to share to help others?

Acknowledge emotion: It is very common to experience anger and frustration following the event that damaged the brain. These emotions could be caused by injury to the parts of the brain that control emotional expression. They could also be due to frustration and dissatisfaction with changes in life brought on by the injury (loss of job, physical abilities, and independence). Some people struggle with being isolated, depressed and/or misunderstood.

Acceptance of my new life and limitations was the starting point to embracing the new me. Different can be good. I find that being perfectly imperfect is far less stressful. Previously, I was so goal oriented that I lived life always on a mission. If I passed you on the street, I would politely say, "Hi" but my head was busy focusing on the goal I was trying to accomplish and that was where my thoughts were focused. Now, holding onto a thought or a goal is often fleeting. This frees my mind to welcome conversations with family and friends. I feel much more connected within my circle now. I love this part of the new me.

Another part of acceptance was giving myself permission to let go of the old me. I had to replace the anger of "I can'ts" with celebrating the "I can's" and be excited about discovering the new me. I had to affirm to myself that I wasn't giving up, I was letting go of the things I couldn't change. I regularly take stock of how far I've come, express gratitude for these successes, and acknowledge that I am perfectly imperfect and that's okay.

Gratitude is HUGE. Although it felt so fake at first, I really did have to "Fake it till you make it." Once I recognized that I was dwelling in a space of victimhood, one of the small steps I took to crawl out was finding things I could be grateful for. Initially small items of gratitude like having a warm blanket, the feeling of freshly brushed teeth and being able to figure out the TV remote began to evolve into more significant moments of appreciation. Grateful to have Blair's support, grateful to have found audio books and other educational audio resources, grateful to have very little residual physical impairments, grateful to relearn tasks even if the learning is temporary.

Sleep is incredibly important. I want to get the best sleep at night that I can. Also, when I have times of extreme fatigue due to too many mental challenges or exceptionally emotional events, it is important that I nap (whether it is for 20 minutes or 2 hours). I'll wake up when my brain is ready to go again. I've also learned to educate people in my social circle that there is the possibility that I will need to "rest."

We can then make accommodations for a quiet space, if needed. Being able to comfortably set up boundaries took a while for me, but became easier as people become more aware of my needs.

Asking for help is becoming so much easier. I think being uncomfortable in this area in the past had a lot to do with my ego. I would define ego, in this instance, as the part of "self" that is tied to my occupation, my educational background, my financial status and my abilities. When these are taken away, you are stripped to the core of who "self" really is. Losing all those things was hard. I felt angry and lost for so long. I wanted "the old me" and my old life back. Once I accepted these parts of "me" were gone, I was pleasantly surprised to find that at the very core of "me" resides a caring woman that is energized by helping others. A woman I am proud of.

Power to choose. Event plus reaction equals outcome. It isn't always easy, but you have the power to choose how you respond to every life experience. You can choose your attitude. This has been the most valuable equation I've learned. When I get overwhelmed, I make my best effort to stand back, take a look at what's going on as though I was looking at someone else's life, and then choose how I'm going to react.

Faith. Throughout this experience my faith has remained strong. I believe with all my heart and mind that God loves me more than I can comprehend. I honestly believe that everything that has happened in my life has happened for me and not to me. Even through the months of anger and frustration, I remained curious about God's purpose in this experience. I see the blessings now. I've been given more time at home with Blair, watched my relationships with family and friends grow, I've found new ways to keep my inquisitive mind satisfied—I've even enjoyed walking more. Maybe it's this faith that gives me hope that my new life will be exactly what it's meant to be.

My wish is that sharing my story and struggles will help to encourage others finding their way through the experience of a new brain injury and ultimately provide hope that life can be better. In my case, I went from a terrifying stroke to a life of gratitude, hope, and grace.

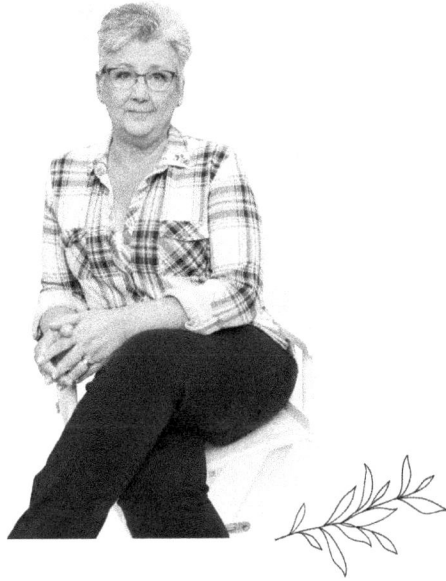

Julianne Heagy

Biography

Born in July, 1958 in Woodstock, Ontario, Julianne Peter was the third of five children born to two very loving, hardworking, entrepreneurial parents. Raised in the small community of Melbourne, Ontario, the author started her schooling in a one-room school and advanced to larger, multiroom schools in Glencoe, Ontario for her middle school years to grade 11.

Being an adventurous child, in her late teens, Julianne hopped on a train to Saskatchewan to help family friends with childcare needs. That began her love of western Canada and eventually she joined the family friends in Fife Lake, Saskatchewan and took her grade 12 at Rockglen School in the neighbouring community. It was there she experienced her first brain injury from a car accident and, incidentally, met her husband, Blair Heagy.

In the following years, her work took her between Ontario and Saskatchewan. Career choices started as a server at Kentucky Fried Chicken, to the secretarial pool at Revenue Canada, then to a lengthy career in insurance, banking, and then as a medical records tech at various local hospitals. From 1997 to 2009, Julianne managed her own retail business that evolved from a gift shop into a day spa (all while she continued to work part-time at local health facilities). In the years that followed, she continued to do remedial massage therapy from her home and work for the health district, finally taking on the position as a Member Relations Officer for a co-operative retail.

Having a natural curiosity, a sense of adventure and an affinity for learning, the author completed many courses and acquired several certifications: Office Education (Saskatchewan Technical Institute); Fellowship of the Life Management Institute with a specialty in Selection of Risk and Information Systems (computers, before they were in every office); Medical Record Technician (now Health Information Manager or HIM); Chartered Herbalist; Registered Massage Therapist; Low Intensity Laser Therapist; and a certificate in Commercial Credit Administration.

www.ingramcontent.com/pod-product-compliance
Lightning Source LLC
Chambersburg PA
CBHW081414270326
41931CB00015B/3273